The Art of Medicine
in relation to
the Progress of Thought

CAMBRIDGE
UNIVERSITY PRESS

University Printing House, Cambridge CB2 8BS, United Kingdom

Published in the United States of America by Cambridge University Press, New York

Cambridge University Press is part of the University of Cambridge.

It furthers the University's mission by disseminating knowledge in the pursuit of
education, learning and research at the highest international levels of excellence.

www.cambridge.org
Information on this title: www.cambridge.org/9781107690295

© Cambridge University Press 1945

First published 1945
Re-issued 2014

A catalogue record for this publication is available from the British Library

ISBN 978-1-107-69029-5 Paperback

The Art of Medicine in relation to the Progress of Thought

A Lecture in the History of Science course
in the University of Cambridge
February 10, 1945

By A. E. CLARK-KENNEDY

M.D., F.R.C.P., *Physician to the London Hospital
and Dean of the Medical School,
Fellow of Corpus Christi College, Cambridge*

CAMBRIDGE
At the University Press
1945

CONTENTS

The Hippocratic period . . . . *page* 7

The Renaissance 14

The last hundred years 16

The new conception of disease . . . 20

Preventive medicine 26

Principles of treatment 31

The mind in relation to disease . . . 35

Medicine and modern life 43

THE
ART OF MEDICINE IN RELATION TO
THE PROGRESS OF THOUGHT

By general consent there are good and bad periods in art. When art is bad, good art does not exist. When art is good, good and bad art flourish side by side. It is the same in medicine, which is sometimes honoured by inclusion in the distinguished company of the arts, and it is to the good medicine in these relatively good periods that we must look to discover the contributions which medicine has made, if any, to the progress of human thought.

I cannot, however, claim any particular knowledge of the history of medicine, and propose to devote most of my time this morning to modern medicine in relation to current thought. Nevertheless, in order to fulfil my task, I must attempt a brief review of the three great periods of the past. The first, or Hippocratic, runs from the sixth century B.C. to the death of Galen at the end of the second century of the Christian era. The second begins with the publication of *The Fabric of the Human Body* by Andreas Vesalius in 1543, and includes the discovery of the circulation of the blood by Harvey, and the work of Mayow and others on respiration and combustion. This period ends for the purpose of this lecture in the seventeenth century with the posthumous publication of the first complete book on the physiology of the human body by René

Descartes, the contemporary and correspondent of the English philosopher, Thomas Hobbes, and with the vitalism of the German physician, Stahl, who also promulgated the phlogiston theory. The third period emerges out of the solid complacency of the eighteenth century and the upheaval of the industrial revolution, and includes Darwin's publication of *The Origin of Species* in 1859, Pasteur's disproof of the spontaneous generation of life, the discovery of the bacterial cause of many diseases, Mendel's work on genetics, and Lister's antiseptic and aseptic surgery. It covers roughly the last hundred years, and culminates in our own day in the discovery of insulin, Pavlov's description of conditioned reflexes, Freud's work on the subconscious mind, increasing knowledge of the viruses and genes, and finally in the discovery of the sulphonamides and penicillin, with the dramatic fulfilment of Ehrlich's dream of chemotherapy.

I am also confronted with an initial difficulty in interpreting my terms of reference as a lecturer in this course. Medicine is not a single science, but depends on the integration of a number of sciences for the specific purpose of understanding the nature of disease as a natural phenomenon, and the application of these and other sciences to the practical problems of the prevention and treatment of ill-health. We are not concerned with the contributions that individual medical men may have made to thought, unless it can be claimed that their particular contributions to science have had an effect on our way of thinking specifically through medicine. Rather,

6

we must consider the way in which medicine, by bringing science and thought into intimate and personal relationship with humanity, has resulted in science making a greater contribution to thought than would otherwise have been the case. Copernicus, a physician, revolutionized our ideas of the universe, but not through his profession. Aristotle never practised medicine, but influenced medicine profoundly, and, through medicine, human thought for over a thousand years.

THE HIPPOCRATIC PERIOD

The Greek physicians of the school of medicine associated with the name of Hippocrates made three great contributions. In the first place they broke away from preconceived ideas, and started to observe disease as an objective phenomenon of nature, keeping records of cases which are remarkable for accuracy and detail. They knew little about the physiology of the body, and less of the causes of disease. Nevertheless, they emphasized the integration of the functions of the body as a whole, and regarded disease as disharmony of the body or mind, an aspect of medicine which was lost sight of until revived by Sydenham in the seventeenth century. But their great achievement was to lay the foundation of the observational method in the study of natural phenomena, and by so doing to make a contribution to science in general, and in consequence to the progress of human thought, which it would be difficult to overestimate.

Secondly, against the corrupt background of temple medicine, in the atmosphere of the declining mythology of the Greek religion, and in the pre-Christian era, they adopted the best moral standards of the age, as reflected in the life of Socrates and the philosophy of Plato, and laid down the ethical code for the practice of medicine which survives to this day. 'I swear by Apollo, the healer, invoking all the gods and goddesses to be my witnesses, that I will fulfil this Oath and this written Covenant to the best of my ability and judgement. I will look upon him who shall have taught me this Art even as one of my own parents. I will share my substance with him, and I will supply his necessities, if he be in need. I will regard his offspring even as my own brethren, and I will teach them this Art, if they would learn it, without fee or covenant. I will impart this Art by precept, by lecture and by every mode of teaching, not only to my own sons, but to the sons of him who has taught me, and to disciples bound by covenant and oath, according to the Law of Medicine. The regimen I adopt shall be for the benefit of my patients according to my ability and judgement, and not for their hurt or for any wrong. I will give no deadly drug to any, though it be asked of me, nor will I counsel such, and especially I will not aid a woman to procure abortion. Whatsoever house I enter, there will I go for the benefit of the sick, refraining from all wrong-doing or corruption, and especially from any act of seduction, of male or female, of bond or free. Whatsoever things I see or hear concerning the life of men, in my attendance on the sick or even apart therefrom, which ought not to be noised abroad, I will keep silence thereon, counting such things to be as sacred secrets. Pure and holy will I keep my Life and my Art. If I fulfil this Oath and confound it not, be it mine to enjoy Life and Art alike, with good repute among all men at all times. If I transgress and violate my oath, may the reverse be my lot.'* There are those still living who were required to take the Hippocratic oath on attaining the University degree which entitled them to practise physic.

In the third place, Greek medicine established the idea of the physician as a necessary aid to living in human society. The legendary figure of Hippocrates has become the personification of the wisdom and experience for which all crave in sickness and anxiety, and of the physician as guide, philosopher, and impersonal friend whom many require even in health. Hippocrates must surely have inspired 'the wise physician' of the unknown writer of Ecclesiasticus, and Luke, 'the beloved physician' of St Paul. If Greek medicine has set an example to which my profession must endeavour to aspire, it has at the same time provided a type behind which, granted the necessary presence and the power to act a part, charlatanism, ignorance, and insincerity, can be successfully and even profitably concealed.

The philosophy behind Greek medicine was characteristic of an age of uncertainty and doubt, and comparable

* The Hippocratic Oath. Charles Singer, *A Short History of Medicine*. Oxford, at the Clarendon Press, 1928.

with that of the Stoics at a later date. The world was designed by God; all events in the natural world were determined by forces outside Man, who had no power to control his destiny. Epidemics came and went with a regularity comparable almost to the return of the seasons and the ebb and flow of the tides. The physician, who could do little for his patient, had to rely on the natural tendency of the body to effect recovery, and advocate patience and resignation. All was for the best, even death. 'The time of man's life is as a point, the substance of it ever flowing, the sense obscure; and the whole composition of the body tending to corruption. His soul is restless, fortune uncertain and fame doubtful; to be brief, as a stream, so are all things belonging to the body; as a dream or as a smoke, so are all that belong unto the soul. Our life is a warfare, and a mere pilgrimage. Fame after life is no better than oblivion. What is it then that we will adhere to and follow? Only one thing, Philosophy. And Philosophy does consist in this, for a man to preserve that spirit which is within him from all manner of contumelies and injuries and above all pains or pleasures; never to do anything either rashly, or feignedly, or hypocritically; wholly to depend upon himself and his own proper actions: all things that happen unto him to embrace contentedly, as coming from Him, from Whom he himself also came; and above all things, with all meekness and a calm cheerfulness, to expect death, as being nothing else but the resolution of those elements, of which every creature is composed. And if the elements themselves suffer nothing by this perpetual conversion of one unto another, that dissolution and alteration, which is so common unto all, why should it be feared by any? Is not this according to Nature? But nothing that is according to Nature can be evil.' *

Aristotle, however, had been brought up in the philosophy of Plato, and had been profoundly influenced by the methods of the physicians. He extended systematic observation to almost the whole of the natural world, dissected animals, arranged them in a natural order, studied their different methods of reproduction, and founded comparative anatomy. He speculated in physiology, came to the conclusion that the heart was the seat of the emotions— Plato had realized that the brain was the physiological basis of the mind—and introduced conceptions which, although largely erroneous, dominated medicine throughout the Middle Ages. His main influence on thought was to correlate Plato's idea of the soul with the physiology of the body. This teaching long survived his death, and when, soon after, the intellectual centre of the world shifted to Alexandria, the first medical school was established on the basis of Aristotle's system of natural philosophy. Herophilus started to dissect the human body, and Erasistratus to speculate more exactly on the different parts which were revealed. Erasistratus, indeed, adopted the materialism of Epicurus, who had revived the atomic

* *The Meditations of Marcus Aurelius*: Second Book, xv, translated by Meric Casaubon. Everyman's Library, No. 9. J. M. Dent and Sons Ltd., 1906.

theory of Democritus, and the stoic philosophy of Zeno, which had dominated Alexander's empire. He admitted the existence of a designing force in nature, but denied the soul which Aristotle postulated, and attributed the peculiar characteristics of living things to some subtle essence which he confused with air and breathing. Nevertheless, the spirit of original inquiry was almost dead, science was already on the decline, and Galen, at whose death in A.D. 200 the classical period comes to an end, made only a few original contributions. But by his voluminous writings as a physician he popularized the conceptions of Aristotle, including his conjunction of Plato's idea of the soul with the physiology of the body, rather than the materialism of Erasistratus. Moreover, he saw in the body greater evidence of design than Erasistratus would allow, and more opportunity for free-will and independence of the human mind than the Stoics would admit. By adopting Aristotle's conception of the relation of the soul to the physiology of the body, Galen helped to prepare the world for the acceptance of the idea of individual responsibility and the Christian interpretation of human life.

The Israelites had introduced the idea of a covenant between Man and a single universal God. The Greek philosophers had argued in favour of an abstract morality, the metaphysical existence of God, and the survival of human personality. These two points of view met in the Hellenistic world. And now Aristotle's conception of the relation of an immaterial soul to a material body, designed by a Creator, was being popularized in the writings of a physician who, although lacking in originality, dominated medical thought throughout the Middle Ages. Galen's teleological teaching was naturally attractive to the protagonists of the new faith, which preached a Trinity of three Persons, individual responsibility, original sin, and redemption by grace. On the other hand, medical science was likely to make little progress in a world in which the human body, where Galen had seen so much beauty and evidence of design, was now largely an obstacle to salvation, and had become the 'vile body' of the Pauline epistle which must be kept under subjection in order to gain salvation. The power of mind over body became greater than at any other period in the history of the world. The saints and martyrs suppressed pain and fear in spiritual exaltation to a degree which has never since been achieved, and the body was deliberately subjected to maltreatment and hardship to be purified of the lusts of the flesh to an extent to which it is now difficult to imagine. It would be interesting to know the incidence of deficiency disease, tuberculosis, and hypochromic anaemia in the cloisters at Tintern, Fountains and Rievaulx, where the Cistercian rule demanded strenuous labour in the fields on a scanty diet, repeated blood-letting, and nightly interruption of sleep to carry out the offices of the Church. It would be still more interesting to know the extent to which depression of the function of the brain, on which mind depends, by the deliberate cultivation of ill-health, influenced the development of theological doctrine, or contributed to a spurious form of individual morality and saintliness. Interest in the body and the power of medicine inevitably declined, as the Church struggled to dominate the declining Empire in the West.

At the Renaissance, the physical and biological sciences were conceived out of art in the mind of Leonardo, who investigated mechanics, and studied anatomy and physiology. The first child, physics, became viable in the work of Copernicus, Galileo, and Kepler. Biology was born second, in the studies of Vesalius, Harvey, and Malpighi: and, ever since then, has limped along behind the mechanical sciences in the part-worn clothes of her elder sister, physics. Copernicus described the revolution of the planets, and Vesalius gave an account of the static structure of the human body. Galileo enunciated the principles of mechanics, and Harvey applied them to the circulation of the blood. Boyle rescued chemistry from alchemy, and Mayow applied chemistry to the physiology of the body. The materialism of Erasistratus was triumphant: Aristotle's conception of the soul and Galenism were dead. The body was a machine which worked by mechanical laws, and consciousness and mind were by-products of the material world. Metaphysics was not yet ready to criticize this point of view. No wonder that the Church reacted so violently, for on the new theory the body was all important, and the soul did not exist. Surgery advanced rapidly, aided by more accurate knowledge of anatomy; modern physiology had been founded by Harvey; and Sydenham

14

started the description of diseases as clinical entities, a limited point of view which persists in orthodox medicine, to some extent, to this day, and still dominates the lay conception of disease. But the physiology of the Renaissance left no room for the soul, and, although Sydenham revived much of the best in the Hippocratic system, the mind was neglected, and medicine, even in the hands of Sydenham, failed to restore the philosophical position.

The reaction against the new materialism was not long delayed. Descartes described the body as a machine, but attributed to man a soul, which he denied to animals, and located the soul in the pineal gland at the base of the brain. This crude conception made no particular appeal, and the more important reactions to the materialistic physiology of the seventeenth century came from Germany, where Stahl, the chemist and physician, introduced the conception of vitalism, maintaining that the particular behaviour of living things was controlled by vital laws which were entirely different from the laws which governed matter. The metaphysical controversy was now well started, and dominated the thought of the eighteenth and early nineteenth centuries, although Locke, Berkeley, Hume, and Kant made little contribution to thought which the ordinary man could understand. Medicine certainly made no particular contribution to metaphysics, but during the eighteenth century progressed rapidly on the foundations laid by Sydenham. Throughout this period, medicine cannot claim to have made any particular contribution to human thought.

Meanwhile, the microscope had been perfected, and during the first half of the nineteenth century Schwann and Schleiden showed that the smallest unit exhibiting the peculiar characteristics of life was the single cell. On this basis Virchow founded his cellular pathology of the human body. In 1859 Darwin published *The Origin of Species*, and almost in the same year Pasteur disproved the conception of the spontaneous generation of life, demonstrated the specific chemical action of ferments, and proved the bacterial origin of certain diseases. In 1900 the work of Mendel, Abbot of Brünn, was rediscovered, De Vries described mutation, and Planck introduced the quantum theory, although the fundamental interrelationship of these discoveries is only now beginning to be realized. The science of genetics was developed, and the discovery of the chromosomes provided the anatomical basis for the new theory of heredity. Conditioned reflexes were investigated by Pavlov. Heredity soon became a matter of accidental reshuffling of genes, and behaviour a succession of conditioned reflexes. Practical medicine had also made great advances. Antisepsis and asepsis reduced the mortality in surgery, and the introduction of anaesthetics abolished the horror of the operation. But on the philosophical side the pendulum was swinging back in the direction of materialism and determinism in biology, and once more science came into conflict with the Church.

Although evolution was now certain, Darwin's theory was far from satisfactory, and much still remained to be explained. Haldane at Oxford revived the vitalism of Stahl, but we are gradually beginning to realize that biology has been working on a system of physics already out of date. Energy and matter have become different aspects of one reality, which man, limited by the structure of his brain and mind, can only conceive as electrons charged with energy moving in human concepts of space and time, and which the mathematicians describe as quanta in a four-dimensional space-time continuum. The law of conservation of energy is now merely a restatement of the law of conservation of matter, and it is doubtful if the human mind is capable of understanding the nature of the physical universe. But if the distinction between energy and matter has ceased to be absolute, that between living and non-living things until recently at least still seemed to hold. Nothing exhibited the criteria of life which did not possess some organized structure. Now, the viruses, which are the cause of such diverse conditions as the bacteriophage phenomenon, mosaic disease in the tobacco plant, the common cold, measles, infantile paralysis, and chicken-pox and small-pox, have been shown to vary in size between the smallest bacteria and the larger molecules. The smaller viruses can hardly possess organic structure, as ordinarily understood, although some can be obtained in a crystalline state. Chemists still endeavour to think of them as molecules. On the other hand, they increase and multiply in number, and bacteriologists still try to regard them as cells. They have not appeared where they were not known to exist before, and so far have only been found, and can only be cultivated, in association with living cells, which probably provide the enzyme systems necessary for their existence. The exact significance of the viruses in relation to living cells and inorganic molecules still remains to be determined.

The smallest viruses are comparable in size and possibly of similar nature to the genes, which, although limited in number, provide in the fertilized ovum the genetic plan and the motive force leading under favourable environmental circumstances to the full development of the individual. The genes are now regarded as being of the size of large molecules, and a physicist* has recently pointed out an important implication of this discovery. The ordinary laws of physics are statistical laws which are only valid for large accumulations of atoms or molecules. Each molecule or ion moves differently in the diffusion of a gas or the solution of a solid. The human body is of a sufficient size to be influenced by accumulations of matter large enough to obey the statistical laws of physics with a considerable degree of accuracy, and to be immune to the behaviour of individual molecules in the environment. The gene is a relatively small collection of about a million atoms, too small an aggregation to obey the statistical laws of physics, and yet the genes have succeeded in transmitting the main hereditary characteristics of the human species

* Erwin Schrödinger, *What is Life?* Cambridge University Press, 1944.

practically unchanged through hundreds of thousands of years. The explanation lies in the fact that the gene is a molecule in which the atoms are arranged in the non-repetitive structure of an aperiodic crystal. In a molecule of this kind, there are only a certain number of possible stable configurations without intermediate states. The transition from one configuration to another takes the form of a quantum jump, and demands the application of the appropriate form of energy. On the one hand, therefore, the genes have tended to remain unchanged, and have exerted a constant heredity effect down the ages, in spite of the fact that they are too small to obey the statistical laws of physics. On the other, the application of X-rays in sufficient quantity will produce mutation in the germ plasm in a degree proportional to the amount of radiation to which the germ plasm is exposed. Mutations thus produced are transmitted according to the laws of heredity to subsequent generations derived from the particular cell in which the mutation was produced. There may be little difficulty in supposing that the structure of the aperiodic crystal constituting the gene is sufficiently complex to provide a specific pattern corresponding to the hereditary characters which it transmits. The mechanism by which this pattern in the fertilized ovum is translated into action, and results in the full development of the individual, is entirely another matter, and remains at present altogether unexplained. For life creates form and structure, and then resists change, and tends to maintain the form and structure which has been created. According to Schrödinger, life resists maximum entropy, and maximum entropy is death. The absolute laws which determine the development and maintenance of life, and which remain to be discovered, may well prove to transcend in importance the statistical laws of physics.

THE NEW CONCEPTION OF DISEASE

Our conception of the nature of disease has changed as knowledge has advanced. The Greeks, who knew practically nothing about physiology, regarded ill-health as disharmony of the body or the mind. During the Renaissance period, it must have seemed more like something wrong with the human machinery, on which the work of Vesalius and Harvey had thrown so much light. In the seventeenth century, Sydenham attempted to classify diseases as clinical entities, an idea which has proved useful in many ways, but has tended to obscure the real nature of disease and often led to a superficial attitude towards the problems of medical practice. As the result of modern discoveries, however, we now know considerably more about the physiology of the body and the psychology of the mind, and although the relationship between body and mind remains almost as obscure as in the days of Plato and Aristotle, we are now able to see man more clearly from the point of view of the physical and social environment in which he lives. In consequence, we are able to form a clearer conception of the real nature of disease.

The body can be regarded as a physico-chemical machine, which has evolved as the result of variation and natural selection in the struggle for existence. No two people are quite alike, because the development of each individual depends on the genetic structure of a fertilized ovum, which provides the plan, and upon the environment, which supplies the materials for its execution. A faulty environment may lead to modification of the accomplishment of the original genetic plan, and an abnormal genetic plan usually leads to an imperfect finished product. This results in a considerable degree of natural variation in the human species. The mind, which can control the body within certain limits, is more difficult to understand, and unfortunately the word 'mind' is used without any precise meaning by many writers. In ordinary conversation we talk about the conscious and subconscious mind with the result that consciousness and mind are frequently confused.* It seems simplest to think of mind as action in the nervous system. According to this definition, mind consists of the passage of impulses in the nervous system, in the same way that the beating of the heart is made up of the contraction of muscle fibres in the walls of the auricles and ventricles. Mind, as thus defined, starts in, and develops with, the evolution of the nervous system, and works in the first instance at the reflex level. There is nothing more mysterious from the physiological point of view about the working of mind, as thus defined, than there is anything peculiar about the action of the heart. The real

* For pointing out to me the common confusion between mind and consciousness, I am indebted to my colleague Dr J. T. MacCurdy of Corpus Christi College, Cambridge.

21

mystery is now consciousness, which makes us conscious of the problem. At some point in organic evolution, consciousness must have gradually or suddenly appeared. We are only absolutely certain about consciousness in ourselves, and our own experience of our own consciousness supplies abundant evidence of the existence of the half-forgotten realm of memory and the working of the subconscious mind. Moreover, we also know from our own experience that the conscious mind can only really attend to one thing at a time, that sensory impressions can be stored in memory, and that the use of muscles laboriously acquired by conscious practice for a certain purpose can, in the process of time, be transferred to the subconscious, and in some cases, as in swimming, to the still lower reflex level of the mind. Behaviour is an unreliable index of consciousness, particularly in animals and in patients under light anaesthesia, in whom co-ordinated movement, and even the outward expression of emotion, may be carried out at the reflex level independently of actual conscious experience. But at some point in development, every human being becomes conscious, as in coming round from an anaesthetic, making pain inevitable, and, as most people believe, some degree of free-will, and some capacity for deliberate thinking, and moral and aesthetic judgment possible. We do not know if mind and consciousness, as thus defined, are merely products of the development of the nervous system, or are the manifestation of something introduced or some force acting continuously from without. All three may be required to explain the evolution of individual character and personality. Nevertheless, the limit of the potential development of the mind in the body, or of the manifestation of mind through the body, seems to be set by the anatomy and physiology of the brain, in the same way that the power to increase the circulation of the blood during exercise, and run long distances, depends on the anatomical structure and physiological efficiency of the heart. Within these set limits, the development of mind depends on the psychological environment, just as the growth of the body depends on the physical environment. Once mind has developed, it exercises a direct effect on the body in two ways. At the higher level of the nervous system, the processes of conscious or subconscious thought can control the skeletal muscles and inhibit reflex action to a considerable extent through the somatic nervous system. Conscious or repressed emotion influences visceral function through the autonomic nervous system.* Conversely, the conscious mind, which depends on the anatomy and physiology of the brain, is profoundly influenced by the physical condition of the body, as, for example, in the delirium of an acute infection, in the 'jaundiced' mental outlook of some minor disturbance of physical health, or in the depression of an attack of influenza. Even the

* The peripheral nerves leaving the central nervous system can be divided into two groups: the somatic and the autonomic. The somatic supply the skeletal muscles which are to a large extent under voluntary control. The autonomic supply the heart, intestine, blood vessels, sweat glands, etc., and are activated by emotion with the result that the physiological condition of the body is adapted to the requirements of the emotional state of the mind as in preparation for action in response to the emotion of fear.

23

instinct of sex is dependent to some extent on endocrine secretion.

The duration of life depends, as far as we can see, on the genetic equipment with which we are endowed, the way in which we live our lives, and our environmental luck; in the same way that the 'life' of the tyre of a motor-car is determined by the initial quality of the rubber, the care of the driver, and the variable state of the roads. There are no absolute criteria of physical or mental health. Disease must be regarded as some departure from average anatomical structure, or an abnormal degree of failure of physiological function, or some reduction of psychological efficiency, due either to adverse factors in the genetic endowment of the individual, or to the misuse of his freewill, or to adverse factors in the environment in which he lives, or to some combination of these causes. Abnormalities of structure and function are sometimes transmitted in a recognizable form through several generations. More often, they result from unfortunate interaction between the genes, derived from the two parents, which combine to produce an unsatisfactory genetic plan. This leads inevitably, as growth proceeds, to mal-development of structure or disorder of function, and if the growth of the brain is involved in this way, the subsequent development of the mind, which depends on the structure of the brain, is bound to be affected. The free-will, with which we believe ourselves to be endowed, can be used to increase or diminish the risks which we run in the environment in which we live. These include physical injury, a diet inadequate to maintain health, chemical poisoning, and infection by the parasites, bacteria, or viruses in nature. The cause of malignant disease and the explanation of the degenerative changes of advancing age have not yet been discovered, but both these conditions are probably due to a combination of genetic and environmental factors. When disease develops rapidly, the patient runs the risk of being overwhelmed before the natural inborn defences of the body can be mobilized. If, on the other hand, disease develops sufficiently slowly, integration of structure and function may be maintained for a while, by a process of adaptation to the changes in the body, with the result that the patient does not complain of symptoms in the first instance. From the point of view of early diagnosis and treatment this may be unfortunate. But sooner or later the internal environment tends to change more quickly, whenever function is overtaxed, and then symptoms supervene. The efficiency of the organism in respect of life in the external environment now gradually declines. Finally, disintegration of the structures and functions of the body results in permanent change in the internal environment, with rapid increase in symptoms. Death ultimately supervenes, first of the organism as a biological unit, and then of the individual cells which in the course of evolution have come to depend on the functional efficiency of the body as a whole. The manifestation of mind inevitably ceases with the breakdown of the physiological functions and anatomical structures of the nervous system. But whether certain aspects of the conscious mind derived primarily from without, or produced during life as the result of action in the nervous system, continue to exist independently of the physico-chemical machinery of the body after death, remains, from the point of view of scientific evidence, at present undetermined.

The prevention of disease must, therefore, be considered from three points of view: genetic endowment, education and the use of free-will, and the control of environment. Diseases of hereditary or genetic origin are difficult to prevent in human society as at present constituted. The eugenic control of birth and marriage hardly seems to be a practical proposition except on a limited scale, and the modification and correction of the accomplishment of a faulty genetic plan by the control of environment is only a theoretical possibility except in certain simple cases in experimental genetics. On the other hand, the incidence of disease due to adverse factors in environment can be considerably reduced by the control of the conditions under which we live. The risks of physical injury on the roads and chemical poisoning in industry are lessened to some extent by traffic regulations and factory legislation. The basic national diet can be influenced through food supplies and the control of income levels, and deficiency disease and malnutrition prevented except in cases of individual neglect, stupidity, or ignorance. The chance of actual infection can be reduced by the control of the distribution of food and the recognition of human and animal carriers. It is impossible to eliminate the risk of infection entirely, but individual resistance can be raised by protective inoculation. Susceptible children can be immunized against diphtheria, most people are protected against smallpox by vaccination, and soldiers are inoculated against the risks of typhoid and tetanus. But in this country, although adequate sanitation can be enforced by law, protective inoculation has never been compulsory, and the individual is free to remain a potential danger to society. Education is necessary to insure that free-will is used in such a way that the opportunities of a controlled environment are employed to secure the maximum degree of physical health and the most successful development of personality within the limits set by the genetic endowment of the body and the developing structure of the brain. Propaganda in relation to health, however, is not without danger. It may aggravate the anxiety of the naturally fearful person, and interfere with the health of the body through the autonomic nervous system. While some people need frightening into taking more care of their health, there are others who would do well to live more dangerously, and many could even afford to let their children do the same!

The maintenance of law and order, a satisfactory economic system, international co-operation, and the prevention of war, are all necessary, if the highest average national and international standards of physical health are to be achieved. The full development of human personality in a modern Utopia is less certain. Ordinary experience of life, and the pages of history, reveal only too clearly that, while minds cannot develop to the full under unsatisfactory conditions, a certain amount of stress, strain, and risk is necessary for the maximum development of human character. Unless human nature changes, however, perfect environmental conditions, even if they can ever be achieved, are not likely to persist. Nevertheless, we can work for improvement in moral and intellectual standards, on which the maintenance of satisfactory conditions of life ultimately depends, and in the meantime more could be done to maintain a higher average level. But while, on the one hand, conditions of life in the environment may be much too bad and the risks in the environment far too great, we know that under certain circumstances life can be too comfortable to promote health, and too soft for the development of personality. Moreover, the elimination of all risk would seriously curtail individual liberty and freedom.

Considerations of this kind raise the problem of the meaning of life, and this is a question from which the practice of medicine cannot altogether escape. There will always be some, like the Stoics, who accept life at face value and ask no questions: 'Nothing that is according to Nature can be evil.' But the majority of people adopt some position between two extreme philosophies. On the one hand, there are those who look for a perfect heaven on earth, and on the other, those who live in hope of a perfect earth in heaven. The protagonists of heaven on earth, like the Epicureans, live life for life's sake. Environmental conditions must be perfect, pain, suffering and disease abolished, social inequalities levelled, and war eliminated: all are futile and serve no useful purpose. Those who live in hope or certainty of heaven regard human life as preparation for a more exalted existence at a later stage. Pain, disease, frustration and war are all part of a training which life provides. These could be reduced to some extent by the growing power of science, or if the neighbourliness of man can be increased, but perhaps they should not be abolished altogether. To the former, life is lived as an end in itself: it is productive of nothing in particular, and has no ultimate significance. To the latter, life is maintaining or manufacturing something. Philosophies of this kind have dominated the great religions of the world, and inspired individual lives. According to Plato, the main object of life was to perfect the soul which came into conjunction with the human body at birth. The Lama in *Kim* went about trying to acquire merit, while the Mohammedan lives life in the hope of a material reward in heaven. According to orthodox Christian doctrine, the world is a place in which individual souls are developed under the conditions imposed by the body for the final purpose of union with God in eternal life. To the less orthodox the object of human existence is the production of souls, which survive death, out of human minds based on matter. The moral philosopher thinks of life as productive of abstract realities such as ultimate goodness, perfection, or unity. Artists and poets interpret life in many ways. For Shelley, expelled from Oxford for atheism, life was creating beauty which, in the well-known words of Keats, is also truth. The majority of our patients have no fixed belief or conviction. Few have thought to any great extent, and many have given up the problem of human life as incomprehensible. Most, however, seem to retain a feeling, born perhaps of the environment which they have 'inherited', that there is some purpose in life, and that life must be lived accordingly. Even the most materialistic usually admit the existence of absolute moral standards and aesthetic values apart from their own environmental background and the biological requirements of life in human society. Medicine does not attempt to choose between these two philosophies, and without being conscious of the fact, adopts a compromise. On the one hand, we stand committed, in consequence of the way in which medicine has evolved out of the medicine of ancient Greece, to the prevention and relief of suffering, without taking into account the possible moral value of pain in the development of character and personality, and to the principle of professional secrecy and individual service to our patients as laid down in the Hippocratic oath. On the other hand, medicine adopts the Christian standards of ethics, and works within civil laws based on Christian standards, and is therefore pledged to the principle of prolonging life under all circumstances, even when this is contrary to the interests of the State, or likely to increase in the end the total suffering of the individual. A man may not commit suicide, either in civil law or Christian ethics, but he is not bound to have an operation to save his life. Nevertheless, we may feel under a moral obligation to advise an operation, if thereby the patient's life can be prolonged, even though his life has long ceased to be worth living for ordinary human reasons. On the other hand, we do not usually hesitate to relieve pain to varying degrees by the administration of drugs, even if this clouds the mind and shortens the life of the dying man, and we do not feel bound to go out of our way to keep a deformed infant alive at birth. At the moment, we are free to exercise our own individual judgment in these cases, and in taking decisions of this kind, we are clearly under a moral obligation to ascertain and meet the wishes of rather than inflict our own ideas upon our patients. The law is not likely to intervene under these circumstances, and the law changes slowly. But it must be remembered that, if at some future date the medical services of the country are organized by the State, these problems may assume more difficult proportions.

PRINCIPLES OF TREATMENT

When a disease has become established in the body in consequence of adverse factors in the genetic endowment of the individual or in the environment in which he lives, the treatment of the condition has to be considered from two points of view: the alteration of normal anatomical structure or disorder or physiological function which is responsible for the patient's symptoms, and the primary underlying cause of the condition. The disorder of function can often be relieved by altering the external environment in which the patient lives. A child with congenital mal-

31

formation of the heart may remain free from symptoms under the care of a special school for children handicapped by this defect, and an adult with early heart failure may be able to undertake some lighter form of occupation without physical distress. In many cases the internal environment of the body can be altered in such a way as to stimulate or depress physiological function according to the requirements of the patient. Digitalis from the foxglove increases the efficiency of the heart; opium from the poppy, bromides out of the ground, and derivatives of barbituric acid from the 'lab', all depress the higher functions of the brain. Sometimes the body can be kept permanently supplied with an active principle which the system cannot produce in sufficient quantities, as in the treatment of cretinism and myxoedema with thyroid, diabetes with insulin, and pernicious anaemia with liver extract.

The treatment of the underlying cause of the disorder of function is often more difficult, but there have been some remarkable advances in this direction in recent years. When disease is due to the persistent action of adverse factors in the environment, as, for instance, lack of vitamins in the diet or chemical poisoning at a factory, some alteration of the conditions under which the patient lives or works in a particular respect is clearly necessary. If, however, disease is actually established in the body, other methods must be adopted. Most cases of infective diseases recover spontaneously on account of the natural reactions of the body, which alter the internal environment in favour of the tissue cells, and against the organisms causing the disease. Sometimes these reactions take place too slowly, and the underlying principle of active immunization against diseases such as typhoid and tetanus depends on stimulating these natural reactions in anticipation of possible infection at a later date. Serum therapy consists, in the same way, in reinforcing the natural defences of the body, as soon as the diagnosis of certain diseases has been established. In diphtheria the bacilli are only found in the throat, while the toxins responsible for the main symptoms of the disease circulate in the blood. The body reacts by altering the internal environment by the production of antitoxin. This process may be too slow, and many lives are now saved by the massive administration of diphtheria antitoxin 'prefabricated' by laboratory animals. The presence of diphtheria bacilli in the throat then ceases to be important, except that the patient may remain a carrier of the disease, and infect other people. In other conditions the internal environment of the body may be altered in favour of the tissue cells by chemical means which may, or may not, subsequently prove to have their counterpart in nature. The best example of this method is afforded by the treatment of pneumonia, meningitis and septicaemia with sulphonamides. Moreover, the recent practical application of the discovery that the fungus *Penicillium* produces a chemical substance, with an adverse effect on colonies of bacteria in the neighbourhood, has raised new possibilities in this direction. The cells of a malignant growth are more sensitive to X-rays and the γ-rays of radium on account of the nature of their metabolism than the cells of normal tissue. This margin, though narrow, is sufficiently great to allow the destruction of neoplastic cells by radiation without damage to the surrounding tissues in many cases, but it is not impossible that chemotherapeutic agents in the treatment of malignant disease will be discovered in due course. The average duration of human life has been prolonged to a considerable extent already by the prevention and treatment of infectious disease by these methods, and by the earlier diagnosis and treatment of cancer along these lines. At present there is no known method of inhibiting the degenerative processes in arteries, which are frequently associated with high blood pressure, and seem to be the main factor in the pathogenesis of the physical changes of advancing age. Nevertheless, progress in this direction is not impossible, although the full consequences of the prolongation of physical life on the continued existence of the mind cannot be foreseen. The unicellular organism and the germ plasm are potentially immortal. Only the multicellular organism, in which the cells have become dependent on each other, exhibit the biological phenomenon of death.

Medicine is much more complicated than Sydenham supposed. Diseases are not specimens like birds and flowers which can be labelled and classified, but complex reactions between the genetic structure of the individual, the free-will with which we believe him to be endowed, and the environment in which he is compelled or elects to live and work. Progressive disease leads to a process of gradual disintegration of the structures and functions of the body, which must be regarded as the reverse of the changes which characterized the development of the individual, and the evolution of the race. Pathology overlaps ecology. When we treat disease, we interfere with the equilibrium of nature. Not only does the human body respond to diphtheria toxin in the circulation by the production of antitoxin, but bacteria causing disease in the body develop resistance to sulphonamides and penicillin with the result that these drugs cease to have their 'normal' therapeutic action. There is always the risk that the elimination of one disease may provide the opportunity for another, and chemotherapy often interferes with the physiological functions of the body. Every advance in medicine creates a new problem in medical practice, education, and administration. If a comprehensive medical service is to become free and available to all, and is not to be abused, it is essential that the general public, and those responsible for the organization of the medical services of the country, should be better informed on the problems of medicine than they have been in the past.

THE MIND IN RELATION TO DISEASE

Nevertheless, the conception of disease which has been outlined, and the brief account which has been given of the prevention and treatment of ill-health are neither as yet sufficiently complete. For, hitherto, we have only considered physical factors in the environment acting on the body, which, if they happen to affect the structure of the brain, must modify the development or influence the working of the mind. In addition, we have assumed the power of free-will to control human life and action in the world in which we live. But the environment may also influence the mind directly through the organs of special sense, and produce emotional reactions which have a profound influence on the physiology of the body through the autonomic nervous system. It must also be obvious that the power of the will depends not only on the genetic structure of the brain,* but also on the psychological environment which a man 'inherited' in childhood, the religion in which he was brought up, the education which he received, the stratum of human society into which he happened to be born, and the moral and intellectual standards of the age in which he lives. Nevertheless, common sense allows every individual a modicum of free-will which enables him to rise superior to circumstances, break tradition, defy convention, or exercise moral, aesthetic or intellectual judgment. On the other hand, Pavlov's work on conditioned reflexes and modern psychology both tend to attribute the reactions of the mind to past or present environmental causes, abolish free-will and the power of deliberate judgment, and reduce behaviour to a succession of reactions which, if the whole complex past psychological experience of the individual could be unravelled, would show that all his behaviour was in fact predetermined from the start.

* At present it is impossible to conceive of the inheritance of mind except through the structure of the brain. Mind may, however, be inherited by some other mechanism of which at the moment we have no conception.

The psychologist endeavours to explain defects in the development of personality, intellect, and character entirely on the basis of the genetic structure of the brain and previous experience in the environment. If the genetic endowment of the individual is poor, as evidenced by a family tendency to mental instability, or the environment in early life unfavourable, the personality, instead of developing under the stimulus of education, may cease to progress, and the expansion of the mind gradually become arrested. Instead of opening out, the adolescent becomes introverted, and his emotional reactions so impoverished that circumstances which would cause grief, pain or pleasure to a normal person may cease to have any particular effect. His personality now slowly disintegrates, the intellectual functions of his mind deteriorate, and the most severe cases end in complete dementia or mindlessness. Another individual develops normally, and passes successfully through adult life, but as the past expands, and the future contracts, he may fail to adapt his life to the unforeseen misfortunes, disappointments, declining physical capacity, and narrowing environment of advancing age. Still handicapped by the genetic structure of the brain, with which he was endowed at birth, the ageing man retires into a world of his own, loses his affections, and becomes peevish, irritable, and selfish, spoiling the life of the younger generation. The intellectual attributes of his mind may be little affected at the start in striking contrast to cases of mental instability due to degenerative or inflammatory changes in the structure of the brain. In organic disease of this kind the picture is entirely different. The intellectual functions of the mind fail first, while the emotional reactions are retained; as exemplified in the unwise generosity of Lear, his unbalanced judgment of his favourite daughter, and in his passionate affection and remorse in that last terrible and tragic scene when he enters carrying the dead body of Cordelia in his arms.

The combination of genetic endowment and environmental circumstances is also responsible for the development of personality. The psychoneurotic temperament is particularly important in medicine. In the pathogenesis of this condition, genetic factors, as evidenced by a family history of mental instability, are less in evidence, and environmental circumstances, particularly the early experiences of childhood, seem considerably more important. In people of this type, the sublimation of instinct and conscious adaptation to the difficulties of life does not take place in the normal way, and unsolved conflicts, fears, and anxieties are repressed into the subconscious, where they remain isolated and detached from the general stream and content of the mind. The patient may lose his conscious anxiety and fear, and seems to have escaped from his difficulties, but the isolated complex in the subconscious creates a state of nervousness, mental tension and fatigue. In some cases this condition results in over-stimulation of the autonomic nervous system, and interferes with the general physical health, producing symptoms identical in certain respects with those of organic disease of the body. This similarity between symptoms of organic and purely nervous origin makes clinical diagnosis difficult, and mistakes in either direction are not uncommon. Moreover, the psychoneurotic patient is always peculiarly susceptible to suggestion, because he succeeds in keeping separate in his mind ideas and motives, which in a normal person would inevitably run together. The result is that people of this type are able to repress into the subconscious mind a desire to escape from an unpleasant situation, or a wish to attract sympathy and attention, or even a determination to obtain compensation for a physical injury; and then adopt symptoms which simulate organic disease, and enable them to obtain their original object without being conscious of their own purely selfish motive. Freud's work, therefore, raises the problem of moral responsibility in a disconcerting way. In the first place, the development of personality, and therefore subsequent abnormal reactions to circumstances, may often be partly attributed to the psychological environment in which the individual was brought up, rather than to primary failure of some moral quality, in the same way that a patient under the action of drugs or in the delirium of fever is not responsible for actions which he may commit. In the second place, the motive in the conscious mind, which the patient believes to be the motive for his conduct, is not always the real motive. The primary selfish and antisocial motive may have been repressed into the subconscious, while the apparent motive makes the patient's action respectable to himself and to his friends. A man, who is naturally lazy, may subconsciously exaggerate symptoms due to minor

39

physical ill-health, or actually develop hysterical paralysis, which conveniently keeps him in bed, and leaves someone else to do his work. A 'headache' may provide anyone of this type with a simple method of escaping from an unpleasant situation, and 'heart attacks' in a woman may result in an unmarried daughter being compelled to stay at home to keep her mother company. In time of war a natural fear of military service may be repressed into the subconscious, and rationalized in the conscious mind into conscientious objection. In the religious life wishful thinking may lead to suppression of doubt, and to a degree of faith greater than might have been justified by the intellect alone.

The genetic structure of the brain cannot be altered. On the other hand, abnormal reactions to adolescence can to some extent be reduced by the control of environment, the careful selection of a school, and the choice of a suitable profession. It is also possible that the development of the psychoneurotic personality can to some extent be prevented by careful education and child guidance, where parents have difficulty or are unwise in handling their children. Nevertheless, the treatment of the parents, rather than of the children, often proves to be essential. Some cases of psychoneurosis have been successfully cured by psychoanalysis, which depends in principle on exploring the mind, until the repressed complex has been discovered, and then helping the patient to face his problem in the open. This is a long process. The buried complex cannot always be discovered, and, if found, cannot always be resolved, in the same way that a surgical operation may fail to discover the cause of a disease, or, having discovered, may fail to remove the cause. Moreover, while it is comparatively easy to restore deliberate damage to the body, and sew up an incision, the mind is not so easily reconstituted. Many patients, who have been submitted to psychoanalysis, never have the same confidence in themselves again. Psychoanalysis is also too elaborate to be of general use, and in the majority of cases we have to rely on persuasion and the application of external discipline. This method does not entail any loss of that self-confidence which it is so important to retain.

The modern tendency in psychiatric treatment is moving away from psychotherapy and in the direction of empirical interference with the normal structure and functions of the brain. Hypoglycaemic shock produced by the administration of insulin, epileptic convulsions induced by drugs or electrical stimulation of the cerebral cortex, or prolonged sleep for days under the action of narcotic drugs, seem to benefit many psychotic and psychoneurotic states. Recently it has been found that surgical division of the association fibres of the frontal lobes of the brain has an effect in altering the personality of some mental patients with the result that a number suffering previously from obsessions, depression, or excitement, and requiring continuous supervision and control, are now able to live fairly normal and unrestricted lives.

In the meanwhile, Freudian psychology has naturally attracted wide general interest, and is having an effect on modern thought, education, and our way of life, which extends far outside medicine. The combination of genetics and psychology is essentially deterministic, but does not exclude, and certainly does not disprove, the existence of free-will, or a capacity for moral and intellectual judgment, independent of upbringing, education, and experience. This is sometimes forgotten by the amateur psychologist and teacher who confuses self-imposed discipline and the deliberate control of instinct with the repression of an unresolved conflict into the general content of the sub-conscious mind. He is apt to see the former as a barrier to self-expression and a hindrance to the natural development of personality: an attitude reflected in the exhibitionism of some modern art and literature, and also seen in the reaction against external discipline and tradition which characterizes modern democracy. We seem at times to be in danger of preventing one form of neurosis merely to create another. The deliberate control of selfish motives and instinct, and even some repression in the strict Freudian sense, are probably both essential, if self-discipline is to be maintained, and the minority must accept the decision of the majority, without abnormal reactions, if the con-sequences of extremes in politics are to be avoided. It is probable that psychology, leaving out of account the possibility of something introduced and influencing the mind from without, and tending to ignore the freedom of the will, only gives a partial explanation of the working of the human mind.

The integration of certain sciences for the purpose of the understanding and treatment of disease has therefore made definite contributions at various times to the progress of human thought. Moreover, the practice of medicine touches philosophy at many points. On the other hand, I am not convinced that modern medicine is influencing thought sufficiently, at a time when recent spectacular advances in medicine are creating altogether new problems. Hughlings Jackson* pointed out that increasing differentiation in the nervous system must always be followed by progressive integration. But in medicine we have not been particularly successful in effecting this necessary co-ordination to keep pace with our own modern discoveries which have broadened our front to an almost unmanageable extent. Specialization seems to be undermining the integration of medicine as a whole. Everything except science has long been crowded out of the curriculum. Yet science deals only with those aspects of human experience which are amenable to treatment by the scientific method. In medicine we are bound to deal with human life and experience as a whole, and half the art of medicine is to adopt a reasonable and practical attitude to the unknown. A purely scientific education is inadequate for the profession of medicine, and medical education is losing touch with the humanities at a time when the power of medicine

* See Hughlings Jackson, *Selected Writings*. 2 vols. 1931, 1932. Hodder and Stoughton.

to prolong life, relieve pain, influence endocrine secretion and to some extent instinct, control birth, dominate the mind, and even change the structure of the brain and modify personality, has increased, is increasing, and is likely to increase still further. I am not moving that this power 'ought to be diminished', but merely wish to point out that there is a real danger in this growing power. There always is danger in power. Medicine has certainly not been sufficiently at the disposal of the general public in the past. Nevertheless, I am sometimes nervous of the increasing power of medicine, freed perhaps from independent opinion and harnessed to the State, to control human life through the medical certificate and in other ways, and dominate human minds through the current and possibly fashionable psychiatry of the day. The greater the growing power of medicine, the more often will medicine be confronted by moral issues, and with increasing frequency will problems, now decided mainly on an ethical basis, come to be settled entirely on grounds of medical expediency and judgment. And even in medicine, the interests of the individual may conflict with the welfare of the State.

What is the answer to this problem? For in medicine, as elsewhere, we have no agreed ethical standards, and in politics the principle of individual freedom is in conflict with the demand for increasing State control of liberty. We live in an age in which scientific knowledge has outrun philosophy, narrow specialization is the order of the day, religion has ceased to be a unifying force in education, belief in the Christian revelation seems to have declined, and excessive anxiety over the health of the body has replaced preoccupation with the welfare of the soul. Humanity seems to be travelling through the night without any white line to keep us in the centre of the road. As knowledge widens, we have less and less ground in common, and our views tend to become more and more extreme. To the humanist, who has no interest in science, the penicillin in the fungus, allied to that which grows on our wartime home-made jam, seems almost trivial, until it saves the life of his wounded son, or cures his wife of puerperal septicaemia; and it is so annoying that the world should be made like that. To the scientist and practical man, enthusiasm for the beauty of art may seem affected, until his preoccupation with material things and human suffering widens into a large interpretation of human life. The rift in University education seems to have grown too great. It must grow no greater. The balance of our system must somehow be restored.

The art of medicine is unique in that it alone seems to occupy a middle place. Medicine has to deal with human personality, and human hopes, human fears, and human failings, in conjunction with the material human body which is liable to so many disasters in the physical environment of our existence. In medicine things spiritual and things material are seen together in conjunction with each other, if *only* he possess the 'art', by a neutral, intimate, and, as he should be, unprejudiced observer. I may have an exaggerated opinion of the importance of my own pro-

45

fession, but for the time being medicine could, and medicine should, be the connecting link reconciling the conflicting points of view of the humanities, on the one hand, and the sciences upon the other. A purely scientific education is inadequate for a profession which deals with so close a relationship between mind and matter, and an education in the arts alone is insufficient for minds compelled to live in a material world. Yet philosophy has dropped out of medical education, and the tragedy is that medical education seems to trail along after a 'half-baked' materialism, already out of date, in an age when medicine could, and medicine must, help to integrate the arts and sciences in University education, if our sense of proportion is to be once more restored. Unless this can be done, we run the risk of losing our intellectual balance, and sinking in the sea of our own widening knowledge.

Science looks for a definite answer to a general question. Medicine demands judgment in a particular case. *That* is the difference. Again and again, in our present state of knowledge, we find ourselves adopting Kant's definition of faith; holding something to be true on grounds sufficient for action, although they may not be altogether sufficient to satisfy the intellect. Medicine teaches the necessity for balanced judgment, and that common sense is often a safer guide than the latest theory founded on apparent knowledge of all the facts. Disease is not entirely environmental in origin or mainly genetic, as others would have us suppose. Our wills are free, and our minds capable of development, but only within the limits of our psychological experience and the structure of our brains. Behaviour is not all conditioned reflexes, and not entirely due to deliberate thinking. There is a happy mean between too much repression and too little self-control: too much individual liberty and too little external discipline: too much comfort and too little hardship: too great a risk and too little security; too much pain and too little suffering. Crime is sometimes capable of psychological or physical explanation demanding treatment, and sometimes due to moral failure deserving punishment. Conscientious objection and religious preoccupation are in some cases methods of escape, in others the result of intellectual judgment. The mind and human personality remain mysterious, partly dependent on the structure of the brain, partly determined by psychological experience, but, let it be remembered, medicine has not yet eliminated, and probably never will finally 'debunk' the soul. The extreme view is seldom right. Medicine seems to me to teach that the white line, though faded, obliterated in places, and always difficult to follow, is still to be found in the middle of the road.

Finally, it is not irrelevant to remember that it is one of the privileges of the practice of medicine to handle the biological phenomenon of death, and here we come into closest touch with the spiritual aspects of human life. To the interpretation of this recurrent riddle, medicine makes no contribution, but we can at least exercise judgment, relieve pain within reason, make up our minds when that operation is or is not worth while, and know, in the words of Clough, when to cease to 'strive officiously to keep alive'.* And if, in an age of scepticism and doubt, we are called upon to adopt the Stoic philosophy, and encourage passive acceptance and adaptation to the infirmities of advancing age; and if in the room downstairs, after the individual life is finished, and medicine defeated at the last, we are compelled to advocate quiet resignation to the inevitable phenomenon of death; it need not be in the words of the sombre meditations of the Roman emperor, but in the lovely language of one of our own Cambridge poets:

> He there does now enjoy eternal rest
> And happy ease, which thou doest want and crave,
> And further from it daily wanderest:
> What if some little payne the passage have,
> That makes frayle flesh to feare the bitter wave,
> Is not short payne well borne, that bringes long ease,
> And layes the soule to sleepe in quiet grave?
> Sleepe after toyle, port after stormie seas,
> Ease after warre, death after life, does greatly please.†

---

* Arthur Hugh Clough, *Collected Poems*. 'The latest Decalogue':
    Thou shalt not kill; but need'st not strive
    Officiously to keep alive.

† Edmund Spenser, *The Faerie Queene*, Canto IX, 40. The words are spoken by the tempter, 'a man of hell that calls himselfe Despayre', to the 'Redcrosse knight'. This does not render the quotation inappropriate for the purpose of bringing consolation in the absence of belief in the orthodox Christian doctrine of immortality.

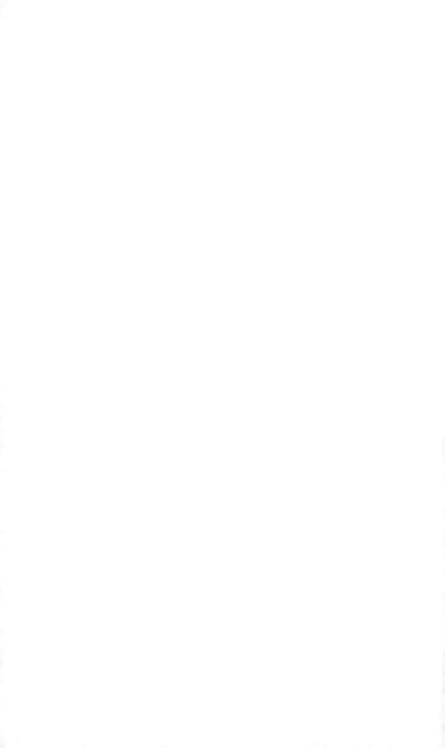

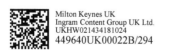

Milton Keynes UK
Ingram Content Group UK Ltd.
UKHW021434181024
449640UK00022B/294